7-Steps to a New Body and a Healthy Lifestyle with Intermittent Fasting

Lose weight, gain confidence and feel great

Dr. Michelle Danville

Disclaimer:

© 2017 – TWK - Publishing. All Rights Reserved.

No part of this publication may be reproduced, stored or transmitted in any form or by any means – electronic, mechanical, scanning, photocopying, recording or otherwise, without prior written permission from the author.

This publication is provided for informational and educational purposes only and cannot be used as a substitute for expert medical advice. The information contained herein does not take into account an individual reader's health or medical history.

Hence, it's important to consult with a health care professional before starting any regimen mentioned herein. Though all possible efforts have been made in the preparation of this eBook, the author makes no warranties as to the accuracy or completeness of its contents.

The readers understand that they can follow the information, guidelines and ideas mentioned in this eBook at their own risk. All trademarks mentioned are the property of their respective owners.

Table of Contents

Introduction

I want to thank you and congratulate you for downloading the book, "7-Steps to a New Body and a Healthy Lifestyle with Intermittent Fasting: Lose weight, gain confidence and feel great".

I was nearing 40, an accomplished woman but was unhappy and no longer confident with how I look. I was fat. It was taking a toll on my self-confidence, and above all, my health.

It was then that a friend told me about Intermittent Fasting. With my busy work schedule, I thought that I couldn't do it. I had my hesitations. I tried many kinds of diet, but nothing worked. So in the end, I committed myself to Intermittent Fasting.

Several years later, I have accomplished more. Aside from that, I've never felt this good about myself. I am fit and feel more confident. I want you to achieve the same. There is no reason to get stuck. I have compiled everything that you need to know about this diet that changed my life forever.

I hope that this helps you in the same way that it helped me become who I am today. Do not feel depressed and get out of your shell. Make this part of your lifestyle now.

Thanks again for downloading this book, I hope you enjoy it!

Chapter 1
Step 1 Education – Why are people getting fat

Junk food is not healthy. This is a common knowledge that many people choose to ignore. Eating too much fast food can cause certain ailments, such as heart problems, high blood pressure, and depression, among others.

Why do you keep on doing something that you know in your mind is wrong? According to Dr. Steven A. Witherly, a food scientist and a leading expert in product formulations and nutrition, eating tasty food is a pleasurable experience. This is caused by two factors. First, the satisfying level that you'll reach will define the sensation of eating. This comes from combined factors that force the brain to associate a sensation with a particular food.

These factors are the orosensation or how the food feels once inside the mouth, how it tastes, and how it smells. The second factor is the macronutrient composition of the food. When it comes to fast food, manufacturers spend money and time in making sure that they'll be able to come up with the perfect blend of fat, sugar, and salt that will excite your brain and urge you to keep on eating, which in the long run, will make you fat.

How do you usually feel after eating too much? Does the food fuel you and give you more energy? This is supposed to be the case if only you'll remember to eat the right type and amount of food per meal. When you eat too much, more blood goes into your digestive system than into the brain. As a result, you will feel sleepy and tired, or it can also be fatal as it can lead to food coma.

Intermittent Fasting

The concept of fasting is not new. You actually do it every day even if you are not aware of it. This is where the term for breakfast was coined. It is the meal that breaks the fast that you voluntarily do as you sleep. Fasting means that you will not eat for a certain period of time. This is quite okay since humans can actually survive without eating for more than three weeks. Fasting is also a religious practice done in Islam, Christianity, and Buddhism. This is also an ancient practice that has been proven to offer health benefits.

Intermittent fasting (IF) requires you to stop eating at irregular intervals for a period of time. It is also an umbrella term used to refer to the various kinds of diet schemes with a cycle that happens in between fasting and eating phase. The different types of IF vary in the covered hours of the eating window and the period of intervals.

There are two types of IF – short-term and long-term.

Short-Term Methods of Intermittent Fasting

12-hour IF

This only requires a little adjustment from your normal diet. This is recommended for people who only want to avoid obesity or lose a little weight.

In this kind of IF, you'll eat 3 meals every day during the hours included in your eating window. You will choose the schedule of your eating window. For example, you can set it from 7 AM to 7 PM, which means that you can eat the 3 meals within this time period. You can no longer eat from 7 PM till 7 AM the next day. Have a light breakfast the next day to break the fast. Avoid taking in too much sugar.

16-Hour IF (Lean Gains)

This requires a 16-hour fasting duration every day. This means that you will have 8 hours for your eating window. Fasting is typically done from 7 PM to 11 AM, which means that you won't eat breakfast since the window falls from 11 AM to 7 PM.

This IF method was further developed by Martin Berkhan and named it after his website, Lean Gains. This is recommended to bodybuilder and people who want to lose fat and build muscles. The fasting period depends on your gender. It is usually 14 hours each day for women and 16 hours for men. It is important that you don't take in calories while on the fasting state but you can have black coffee, calorie-free sweeteners, sugar-free gum, and diet soda.

You are free to choose what time you will begin fasting and in this kind of IF, it typically depends on the schedule of your workout. This way, you can prepare your meals ahead of time. For the days that you won't work out, for example, it is recommended to consume more fat. If your workout is scheduled after fasting, you have to consume more carbs than fat. In any days, your protein intake should be fairly high.

The Warrior Diet

The fasting period for this type lasts for 20 hours, so this is only suited for people who are committed and serious about the program. The fasting period requires you to under-eat so you won't go for 20 straight hours without food. You can eat a little serving of vegetable or fruit. Break the fast by eating a large meal at night.

As opposed to the first 20 hours, you can now overeat during the 4-hour eating window. While you are allowed to eat a lot at this point, you cannot eat food that isn't allowed in the diet. Since you're eating window falls at night, you have to choose food that your body can easily digest before going to bed. Your body will produce hormones from the food that you eat at night, which will be used to burn fat during the day. Make sure that the meal is nutritionally complete. You can add a little amount of carb if you are still hungry.

Long-Term Methods of Intermittent Fasting

Alternate Day Fasting

This requires you to eat only a little for a day and eat like how you normally would the following day. During the fasting period, women should limit their caloric intake to 400 and 500 for men. Do the sequence for the next days until it becomes a routine. Make sure that you don't binge on food when you are allowed to eat. This will defeat the purpose of losing weight. When done right, you can lose up to 2.5 pounds per week by following this kind of IF.

24-Hour IF

This kind of IF has a lot of similarities to the Warrior diet. The fasting period will technically last for 20 hours and you'll have 4 hours of eating window. You will decide what time you will begin fasting. Since you can eat only a meal per day, you can choose to fast from breakfast to breakfast or from dinner to dinner.

This Is recommended for people who are taking medications. You can take your medicines after eating your meal. It is relatively easy to get adapted to this kind of IF. For example, if you have a tight schedule at work, drink coffee in the morning and go about your usual tasks. You can eat dinner upon coming home to get recharged.

Eat-Stop-Eat

This is suited for people who aren't committed to giving up their favorite food but are raring to go on a diet. The practice will teach you a lot about self-control. While you can still eat whatever you want during your eating window, make sure that you take them in moderation.

You will fast for 24 hours once a week. You can do it twice a week after you have gotten used to it. No food is allowed during the fasting period except for calorie-free drinks, but you can eat whatever you like after the fasting period. You can end the fast with a light snack first before eating a meal. You can also opt to eat a complete meal.

This kind of IF reduces your calorie intake, but this won't help you lose weight without exercise. You have to follow a regular fitness routine that includes resistance training.

Go about the process gradually when trying it out for the first time. On your first day, test yourself how far can you go without food. Eat once you feel hungry and stop once you are full. You can add more fasting hours through the days. Fast during the days and hours when you are not busy and you are not required to perform a lot of physical activities.

Fat Loss Forever

Are you the type of person who frequents the gym but always looks forward to their cheat days? This is the kind of fasting that will work for you. It combines the different kinds of IF. This diet requires a 36-hour fasting period, after which, you will follow different protocols of certain IF methods.

Before you can begin with this diet, you need to sign up for a program and follow a 7-day plan. This plan will be based on your gender, age, weight, and how much you want to lose, and the level of physical activities. Make sure that you remain in charge of yourself during your cheat days. Do not give in to your cravings all at once. Eat whatever you want but do it in moderation.

Chapter 2
Step 2 - Find Your Type

There are different adrenal types that can hamper your weight loss goals. How do you get them and what are the reasons why the adrenal glands get burn out? Here are the main causes of the adrenal body type:

1. Taking in high amounts of synthetic ascorbic acid or vitamin C

Naturally, a whole-complex vitamin C is composed of K and J elements, riboflavin, tyrosinase, and an antioxidant element known as ascorbic acid. This means that the synthetic form of vitamin C is composed of only one part. Vitamin C gets stored in the adrenal glands. The latter becomes aggravated when you consume too much of it. You will not feel the side effects early on because the synthetic vitamin C acts as a stimulant. You will realize its downside through the years after it has taken its toll on the adrenal glands. It is best to take whole-complex vitamin C to prevent this from happening.

2. Consumption of adrenal hormones

These hormones come in the forms of steroids or prednisone. Taking them in means that you are taking hormones straight into your body. They bypass the adrenals, which make them weak through time. This does not mean that you must avoid taking steroids altogether, especially when advised by your doctor. You have to be aware that as the steroids affect the adrenals, the tendency is to put on weight.

3. Overwhelming stress

The effects of stress will accumulate through the years. They can drain your adrenal glands, especially if you have been through a lot. Stress is caused by different factors, such as lack of sleep, losing a loved one, too much work, being in the company of stressful people, and many more.

4. Lack of nutrients in the body combined with the consumption of stimulants. Stimulants come in many forms, which include drugs, synthetic vitamins, nicotine, herbal stimulants, appetite suppressors, caffeine, and sugar. These stimulants exhaust the vitamins and minerals in the body. The problem with the adrenal glands gets worse when you are unhealthy and yet you consume too much grains and refined sugars.

5. Infection from viruses, fungus, and yeast

The adrenals are found above your kidneys, so they get a good amount of blood flow. When the causes of infection enter your system, the microbes go along with the blood and get stuck in the adrenals. Through time, the problems will pile up, which will take a toll on the health of the adrenals.

How would you know that your adrenal glands are poorly working? Here are the symptoms that you need to look out for:

- Fatigue and weakness
- Depression
- Sagging and hanging abdomen

- Thinner legs and arms
- Midsection weight
- Need for naps in midafternoon
- Sleepiness
- Can't withstand stress
- Nervousness
- Unhealthy skin
- Red cheeks
- Insomnia
- Dark circles around eyes
- Thinning skin
- Facial hair
- Double chin
- Anxiety
- Full eyebrows
- Round face
- Difficulty getting out of bed in the morning
- Puffy face and eyes
- Patches on the skin
- Reddish stretch marks on the abdomen, arms, thighs, breasts, and buttocks
- Deeper voice
- High blood pressure
- Atrophy of breasts

- Difficulty absorbing calcium
- Asthma
- Ringing in ears
- Chest pains
- Autoimmune problems
- Fluid retention in between cells
- Dehydration
- Low sex drive
- Dullness
- Cravings for sugar, chocolate, salt, and cheese in the evening
- Receding hairline
- Buffalo hump at the lower neck and upper back
- Heel spurs
- Dehydration even after drinking plenty of water
- Fibromyalgia
- Weak bones and ligaments

Chapter 3
Step 3 - Reconditioning Your Thoughts

Your body naturally adjusts to the process when you go into this kind of diet. Train your thoughts to always think positive, especially in the beginning. As much as possible, avoid getting exposed to advertisements that promote food. They will only remind you of hunger and might boost your cravings.

Instead of thinking about food, focus on the health benefits of IF, which include the following:

1. It gives you more energy.

Even when you are not eating, your system burns fat for energy instead of sugar. This is the stored fat that you accumulated whenever you eat in the hours of your eating window. As a result, your metabolic rate increases and you also experience an adrenaline rush.

2. It boosts the secretion of the growth hormone.

The growth hormone increases the fats in the body that it can use as a fuel during the fasting period. It also helps in preserving the muscle mass and the density of the bones. As people age, it is natural that the secretion of this hormone decreases. This leads to weakness and fragility. Fasting serves as a stimulus to push your system to produce this hormone.

3. It lowers your insulin levels.

This will naturally happen when you are not eating. As an added benefit, your system will burn fat, which will lead to the stabilization of the levels of glucose in the blood.

4. Lowers blood pressure

5. Lowers levels of LDL cholesterol and triglycerides

6. Improves cellular repair and turnover

7. Boosts your system's fat-burning capacity

8. Lowers risks of oxidative stress, problems in your lipid, and DNA

9. Improves appetite control

10. Decreases chances of developing cancer

IF improves your overall health. It gives you more energy and enhances your brain function. It is also getting more popular through the years because of its effectiveness in helping people lose weight. It happens as your hormonal levels change. Your body will release norepinephrine, the hormone responsible for burning fat. Even when you only fast for a short period of time, your metabolic rate will increase by up to 14 percent. You will also lose weight because you are consuming fewer calories. In fact, the diet can help you lose about 8 percent of your body weight for 3 to 24 weeks. Among the fats that you will lose, the majority will come from the waist circumference. Aside from looking good, this will result in fewer muscle loss and decreased chances of having related diseases.

Make sure that you monitor the changes in your body at least once a week in the beginning. You will get more inspired to continue with the diet once you begin seeing the changes in your weight and health.

Bear in mind that fasting will not work on its own. It requires your commitment and dedication. You cannot stop once you have achieved your ideal body weight. You have to make this a part of your lifestyle.

Chapter 4
Step 4 - Fat Burner and Non-fat burners

This weight loss diet will not work if you will eat unhealthy food during the hours of your eating window. You can indulge once in a while, but make sure that you always eat in moderation.

Fat-Burning Food

Here are the foods that will ramp up and revitalize your metabolism when you are not fasting:

1. Guacamole

One scoop of this healthy fruit is enough to squash your hunger and speed up the fat burning process. It is rich in monounsaturated fat and vitamin B6. It is a natural appetite suppressant. Many people said that they no longer have the desire to eat for several hours after eating half of the fresh fruit.

2. Cayenne Pepper

This pepper contains capsaicin that helps in boosting the body's capability to turn what you eat into energy. You can add a pinch of cayenne pepper to your favorite dishes, such as eggs, salads, and grilled meats and fish, and start reaping its health benefits.

3. Wild Salmon

This kind of fish is among the healthiest sources of lean protein. Protein helps in developing muscle. Your body will become more efficient in fat burning when it has more muscles. Aside from this, wild salmon also contains a good amount of omega-3 fatty acids. The latter aids in the weight loss process, block the storage of fat, and speeds up the fat burning process.

4. Oatmeal

The whole grains of oats are rich in fiber that keeps you feeling full for a longer duration.

Did you know that eating more than 3 servings of oats and other whole grains per day will give you fewer belly fat than when you eat the same amount of calories from commercially produced white carbs?

5. White Tea

This kind of tea hinders the formation of fat cells or adipogenesis while it boosts the breakdown of your fats or lipolysis. It is also a good source of antioxidants that enables the release of fat from your cells and helps the liver in converting fat into energy.

6. Sweet Potatoes

Sweet potatoes contain slow carbs that make you feel satiated longer. It also gives you more energy even though you are not eating a lot. It contains a good dose of vitamins B6, A, and C. It also has carotenoids that lower your insulin resistance and regulates your blood sugar levels.

7. Berries

Berries boost the fat burning process because they contain polyphenol antioxidants. They also boost the blood flow to your muscles. They are typically used in smoothies and desserts, and are known for being effective in curbing your cravings for anything sweet.

8. Black Beans

These beans contain an insoluble fiber known as resistant starch. It triggers the release of butyrate, a chemical in the system that helps the body in burning fat. They are also a rich source of soluble fiber, which can help a lot in reducing the size of your belly fat.

9. Dark Chocolate

Choose the kinds of dark chocolate with 70 percent and above cacao content. They are rich in polyphenols, a type of antioxidant. The chocolate gets fermented in the stomach, which aids the body in producing polyphenolic compounds that boost fat burning process.

10. Grapefruit

This fruit contains bioactive compounds, the phytochemicals, which help the body in burning fat. It is also effective in suppressing your appetite.

11. Eggs

You can prepare eggs in many ways. They contain a good amount of a nutrient that effectively burns fat, known as choline. Eggs are also rich in lean protein.

12. Pork Tenderloin

When buying any meat, make sure that you get the right cut. A serving of this meat contains 83 mg of choline and 24 grams of protein. This aids in the development of muscles and the reduction of your belly fat, waist size, and BMI.

13. Sun-Dried Tomatoes

They contain two of the most powerful antioxidant: lycopene and beta-carotene.

14. Almonds

These nuts are effective in burning fat. Just by eating 1.5 ounces of almonds per day can help you lose leg and belly fat after 3 to 6 months. It is recommended to eat these nuts before you work out. They contain L-arginine, an amino acid that boosts the carb and fat burning process.

15. Quinoa

This grain has the complete chain of amino acids or complete protein that promotes fat loss and development of muscles. It also contains the highest level of betaine that boosts your metabolism, and a good amount of the amino acid lysine that aids in digestion.

16. Apple Cider Vinegar

It boosts the body's ability to burn carbs. Once the body has dealt with the carbs, it will then face the fats. This will speed up the weight loss process. This vinegar is rich in acetic acid that slows down the flow of sugar in the blood. It also aids in the production of protein that helps in burning fat and in helping you lose weight.

17. Greek Yogurt

Each serving of a 7-ounce cup of this yogurt contains about 20 grams of the muscle-building protein. This is recommended as an after-workout snack because it speeds up the recovery of your muscles. It also helps in fighting off the stress hormone, cortisol, because it has calcium and vitamin D.

18. Grass-Fed Steak

This kind of red meat helps in the development of your muscles. It also prevents inflammation because it contains conjugated linoleic acids and omega-3.

19. Cinnamon

It has polyphenols, the antioxidants that improve your body's sensitivity to insulin. Its main ingredient, cinnamaldehyde, helps you in getting rid of your belly fat. You can add some to your coffee or sprinkle a dash to your oats and other snacks.

20. Lemon Water

Water alone is already an effective appetite suppressant. When you add lemon to water, you will gain health benefits from the D-limonene that a lemon contains. This is an antioxidant found in lemon peel. This kind of water helps in flushing out the fat and toxins from your system.

21. Green Tea

This healthy beverage contains a good amount of the antioxidant ECGC. This aids in the fat burning process and blocks new fat cells from forming. It is recommended to drink up to 5 cups of green tea every day and team it up with a good exercise workout.

This is an effective way of developing toned muscles and in losing fat.

22. Oysters

They are a good source of zinc, a mineral that aids the hormone leptin in regulating a person's appetite. Overweight individuals have lower levels of zinc and higher levels of leptin. When you consume food rich in zinc, your body produces more leptin. You can get 21 percent of your daily RDA of iron from 1/2 dozen of oysters.

23. Cauliflower

This vegetable is thermogenic. It helps your system in burning more calories and in decreasing your body fat.

24. Spinach

It is rich in folate, iron, and Vitamin A. Aside from boosting your energy; it also speeds up the fat burning process. It effectively burns fat due to its thylakoids content. Thylakoid is used as an ingredient in food supplements. Taking 5 grams of this supplement every day can reduce your hunger by up to 25 percent.

25. Spaghetti and Meatballs

You can have a serving of this on your cheat days. Pasta has low glycemic content. It won't drastically change the levels of the sugar in your blood. The meal contains carbs that boost the levels of your leptin that make you feel satiated and also speeds up the fat burning process.

26. Light Tuna

Aside from being affordable, a can of light tuna is a good source of lean protein and docosahexaenoic acid or DHA. You can eat this as a snack, make tuna salad or sandwich. It is also rich in omega-3 fatty acid that boosts the breakdown of fats.

27. Plums

For people who want to lose weight, choose the red plums because they contain more amounts of flavonoids, such as anthocyanins, than the other kinds of plums. They limit the amount of fat that gets stored into your system.

28. Peanut Butter

Look for the brands with the least numbers of ingredients, the most important of all are these two: nuts and salt. Do not buy anything with too many preservatives. The right kind of peanut butter contains monounsaturated fats and nutrients that can make your belly flat.

29. Black Rice

There was a time when only emperors were allowed to eat this rice, which is the reason why it was once called the forbidden rice. This rice is more nutritious than a heaping tablespoon of blueberries. It contains more vitamin E, antioxidants, satiating fiber, and it also has less sugar.

30. Garlic

Garlic contains a compound called allicin, which is responsible for its smell and taste. This compound is also beneficial in fighting off fats.

31. Pumpkin Seeds

The seeds have high levels of magnesium. You can get almost all your daily needs for the mineral by consuming 1/2 cup of the seeds. Your body needs magnesium in order to boost lipolysis and to create and store energy.

32. Cottage Cheese

You can snack on this kind of cheese before going to bed at night. It has high amounts of casein, which is a kind of milk protein and tryptophan, an amino acid that makes it easier for you to sleep faster and deeper.

33. Kimchi

Kimchi, just like many kinds of fermented food, contains high amounts of probiotic. It is unique in a way because of the strains that help in losing and maintaining your weight.

34. Bulgur

This grain is a staple in Mediterranean dishes. It contains satiating fiber, which does not only help you lose weight but keeps your blood pressure regulated. You can add this to vegetables or use as a side dish or a salad ingredient.

35. Jerusalem Artichokes

This root vegetable, also known as sunchoke, is a good source of oligofructose, an insoluble fiber effective in suppressing hunger and controlling your blood sugar levels.

36. Turmeric

This spice contains curcumin, an effective anti-inflammatory nutrient that is also effective in reducing weight.

37. Olive Oil

This is a healthy fat that lowers down the levels of inflammation caused by stored fat.

38. Coconut Oil

This oil is quite effective in helping a person loses weight that there are now several diet programs that use coconut oil as the base or main ingredient.

Non-Fat Burner Food

IF boosts your metabolism and aids the digestion process. Help yourself by avoiding food that will slow your metabolism when you are not fasting. These food include the following:

1. Produce grown on farms that use pesticides and insecticides

While organic fruits and vegetables are not cheap, they also offer health benefits that money can't buy. Consuming ingredients with harmful chemicals will take a toll on your metabolism. According to findings, too much organochlorines in the body, a form of pesticide, will slow down your metabolism and will make it hard for you to lose weight.

2. Refined grains

Refined grains, such as bread, pizza, and pasta, are hard to digest. They also cause extra fat storage and a spike in your blood sugar levels.

3. Too much sugar

Your metabolism slows down when you have high levels of blood glucose. As a result, your body will store more fat and burn fewer calories.

4. Alcoholic drinks

You can have a little amount every once in a while but make sure that you don't take these drinks too often and too much. Alcohol can lead to weight gain. It is also unhealthy for your digestive system and slows down your metabolism.

5. Farmed meats

Always choose the organic type not only when it comes to fruits and veggies but also in meats. Farmed meats are often injected with antibiotics that damage the bacteria in your gut. As it accumulates inside your body, it harms the gut, slows down your metabolism, and makes it easier for you to gain weight.

6. Traditional yogurt

It has a very little amount of probiotic as compared to Greek yogurt. Probiotic are important in maintaining the health of your gut. They reduce your risk of diseases, which include obesity. Read the ingredients of the yogurt before you buy. Stay away with anything that has too much fruit puree and added sugar. To keep safe, choose a high-protein and low-sugar yogurt or 2 percent Greek yogurt with no flavors.

7. Granola bars

They are actually deceiving since they are typically marketed as a health food. These bars may have an oat base that lowers your cholesterol and blood pressure, but they also have a high amount of preservatives, high fructose corn syrup, and sugar. Check the ingredients before you buy one and choose the kinds that do not contain anything that may harm your health in the long run.

8. Frozen meals

These meals typically lack flavors. To make up for what's lacking and to encourage people to try them, these meals are packed with trans-fat, sugar, and sodium. The packaging itself is harmful. Frozen food trays are made of plastic that contains BPA, a chemical linked to gaining weight and in slowing down a person's metabolic rate.

10. Margarine

It is loaded with trans-fats, which slows down your metabolism and makes it hard for you to lose weight.

Intermittent fasting allows your digestive system to rest. It aids in digestion by burning calories and speeding up your metabolic rate. This is beneficial to those who suffer from poor digestion. This will improve your condition and overall metabolic function. IF also improves your hunger and teaches you on how to understand your body when it is really hungry.

Chapter 5
Step 5 - Sleep, Stress, Rest

What do you usually do when you are stressed?

Many people do not only eat but they binge on food, especially when the stress level is too high. What will happen if you are often stressed out? If you will continue your habit of stress eating, it is not impossible to gain a lot of weight in no time.

Many people reach for food when stressed in order to feel better. By satisfying their cravings for anything sweet or salty, the good-mood feelings in the brain get a boost. While this may feel good, you have to realize that it is unhealthy.

You cannot think straight when stressed. Even though you already have planned what to eat, the tendency is to go against it and reach for anything that will make you feel good. The human brain is responsible for controlling the cravings and stress. The neurotransmitters in the brain, such as serotonin and dopamine, control a person's cravings. Your body will control or release these chemicals when you eat something you like or do anything you want. The brains look for these chemicals when you are on a diet. This is the reason why the beginning of the diet is stressful. The diet suppresses the release of dopamine. As a result, you would want to eat more than what you are allowed.

When following any kinds of diet plans, such as IF, always control your mind and not the other way around.

Lack of sleep can lead to overeating.

Sleep deprived individuals tend to put on more calories than those who get enough rest each day. When you lack sleep, your system produces too much ghrelin, a hormone that tells you when you are hungry, and lower levels of leptin, a hormone that tells you that you are full. As a result, you will continue to eat as your body tells you that it is still hungry.

When you are up until late at night, it is hard to control your cravings for snacks. This is an unhealthy lifestyle. You tend to eat small snacks often but don't have the energy to exercise or perform physically tasking activities. This is a common cause of rapid weight gain. When you crave for snacks, you will not go for a celery or carrot. You would want something tasty and loaded with carbs. This unhealthy eating pattern will disrupt your sleep cycle as well.

Make IF Part of Your Lifestyle

Intermittent fasting helps even those who are often sleep deprived. You can adjust your fasting period at times when you are awake and busy with work. This way, you can enjoy your food after you have taken a rest. Make sure that you don't fast after working out. Instead, eat a meal loaded with protein.

Too much stress and lack of sleep and rest can take a toll on your health. Develop the right eating habits and make IF part of your lifestyle. It can help you deal with stress better so that you can avoid eating whatever you like.

Chapter 6
Step 6- Exercise

Intermittent fasting works best when you do high-intensity interval training (HIIT) during your workouts. This kind of exercise helps burn calories in a more efficient manner. The diet will work in eliminating the unwanted weight and fats, which comprise around 65 percent of your body weight. Exercise will work on the remaining percentage by reducing your lean muscle mass.

Choose the easy exercises in the beginning. You have to get used to doing exercises on a regular basis before you go all out with your workout. First and foremost, do not get intimidated. Make sure that you warm up by stretching or walking before you exercise and cool down after by stretching or doing some yoga poses.

1. Pushup

This classic exercise works all parts of the body. It firms up the chest muscles while burning a lot of calories.

Get down with your feet and hands on the floor. Put your hands down in the position that they are a bit wider and parallel to your shoulders. Keep your feet close to each other. Gently move your body down until your chest is almost touching the floor. Push your weight up and go back to the starting pose. Keep your core straight and your hips raised as you repeat the sequence.

2. Cardio intervals

Include the HIIT routine in your workout schedule. Use any cardio equipment that you have – bike, jump rope, elliptical, or treadmill. Follow these patterns for a total of 10 times:

- Give 50% of your maximum strength for 3 minutes.
- Give 75% of your maximum strength for 20 seconds.

- Give 100% of your strength for 10 seconds.

3. Second position plies

This is a common ballet movement. It makes the side of the butt and inner part of the thighs more toned.

Stand with your feet apart. Slightly turn your toes in an outward direction. Bend your knees to lower your body until your thighs are in line with the ground. Put your arms above your head while keeping your shoulders down. Count to three. Gently move your body until you are in your starting pose.

4. Single-leg dead lift

This works on your core and is effective in alleviating back pain. You will need a pair of dumbbells to perform the exercise.

Hold the dumbbells in each hand as your feet stand firmly on the floor. Support your weight with your left foot as you gently lift the other foot. Bend your knee until the lower part of your right leg is in line with the floor. Bend your hips to the front. Bring your body as low as you can handle. Count to three. Gently push yourself back to your starting pose. Repeat the sequence on the other foot.

5. Triceps extension

Use 2-pound weights for the exercise. You can use heavier weights after you have gotten accustomed to the movements. This routine tones your triceps and the back of your shoulders.

Start in a lunge pose and put the back of your heel on the floor. Lean forward towards your bent knee. Gently lift your arms to your side all the way up towards the direction of the ceiling. Put your arms down. Repeat the sequence around 30 times for each side.

6. Shoulder stand

This is a yoga movement that works in reducing your belly fat. Lie down with your back on the floor. Gently lift your hips and legs until your legs are placed above your head. Support your back by placing your hands on your sides. Extend your legs until the line from your ankles to shoulders is straight. Make sure that your neck is relaxed as you hold the pose for a minute. For beginners, you can do the pose beside a wall so you can support your legs with the wall as you hold the pose. Gently lower down your body and legs and go back to your starting pose.

7. Bridge

This exercise is good for the back. It also helps in toning your butt. Lie with your back on the floor. Bend your knees and put your feet flat on the ground. Gently move your hips in an upward direction until you form a straight line from your knees to your shoulders. Count to 5. Gently move your body until you are back to your starting pose.

8. Side Plank

This is a good exercise for the abdomen and is also effective in decreasing the size of your waistline. Lie with the left side of your body on the floor. Keep your knees straight. Use your left elbow and forearm to support your upper body as you move it upwards. Move your hips in an upward manner until you have formed a straight line from your shoulders to ankles. Keep the pose for 30 seconds. Go back to your starting pose and then turn around and repeat the sequence on the other side.

9. Step-ups

This routine strengthens the quadriceps and legs. Put a step or a bench in front of you. Put your left foot on the bench as you push your body in an upward manner with all your might. Stand firm and keep the right foot in line with the left foot. Make sure that your weight is balanced so that you won't fall. Keep your left knees straight as you hold the pose. Lower body and your right leg to the ground. Repeat the sequence on the other leg.

10. Plank with arm raise

This exercise will make you feel taller and more confident. Go into a push-up pose. Bend your elbows and use your forearms to support your weight. Keep the line from your ankles to shoulders straight. Keep your core straight as you raise your right arm to the front. Keep your shoulder blades at the back. Hold the pose then switch your arms.

Remember that exercise is important in this kind of diet. It boosts your energy and tones your muscles. How do you motivate yourself to exercise even at times when you feel like giving it all up?

1. Start slowly. Do not do all the exercises all at once. Pace yourself. Start with the easy movements and increase the difficulty levels of the movements as your body gets used to the routine.

2. Never compare yourself to others. What works for others may not work for you and vice versa. Stick to the routine designed for your body type. You can also modify the exercises if you think that your body is finding it hard to follow the sequence. Through continued practice, your body will eventually get used to the movements and you will find it easier to follow every step of the exercises.

3. Always think positive. Cheer yourself all the time and always think that you can do it no matter how hard it seems.

4. Commit to the program. You won't achieve your weight goals if you will give up too soon.

5. Make the diet and a regular exercise regimen part of your lifestyle.

Chapter 7
Step 7- Stay on the Right Track

Make a plan before you commit to Intermittent Fasting. You also have to create a journal of the steps you have take and the changes that you have observed in your body through time.

You will need to do a lot of adjustments in the beginning. Stay committed no matter what. Fill your kitchen with the right ingredients so you won't be tempted to eat anything unhealthy. Start the diet when you are extremely busy so that you won't have too much time to dwell on your hunger.

By tracking your progress, you will know whether the diet is working or not. What if your chosen method isn't helping you lose weight? You are free to change the method of IF that you are following until you find what works for you.

Here are some more pointers that you have to keep in mind in tracking your progress as you go along the diet:

1. Do not obsess about your weight. Do not expect a big change in your weight for the first few months. Instead of the numbers, monitor the changes in your measurements. Jot them down in your journal. These measurements will indicate your progress as you continue to fast.

2. Check the calorie content of the food and drinks that you consume even when you are not fasting. Also, make sure that you make at least 10,000 steps every day. Monitor your steps by using a pedometer.

3. Monitor fat loss, especially around the waist area. Get your measurements at the end of each week. The right way to measure your weight is by standing with your feet apart. Breathe like usual. Put the tape measure directly against the skin but make sure that it doesn't compress the skin. Get the measurement from the middle part of your lowest rib to the top portion of your hip bone near the belly button.

4. You also have to monitor the changes in the areas of your hips and chest. They are also good indicators whether or not you are slimming down.

5. Aside from the measurements, you must also keep track of your resting pulse rate. Monitor the other health indicators using the right devices, such as fasting glucose, blood pressure, and cholesterol. Frequent your doctor whenever necessary. You have to make sure that you remain in tip-top shape as you go through the diet program. Stop at once when your doctor tells you to.

6. You cannot help other people's comments as well. Take them all in. You can also measure your progress with what they are saying. Aside from your built and weight, they can comment about the other changes that they see in you. Do you look more confident now and more proud of yourself? Do not get easily hurt if you don't believe what other people are saying. Just listen and use all the criticisms to improve and become better.

How do you keep the weight you've lost after reaching your target? Maintenance is necessary for any kinds of diet. IF is no exception. This is the reason why you need to make this part of your lifestyle.

After reaching your ideal weight, you can change the method of fasting that you are following. You can limit the fasting period a day per week. While you can allow more cheat days, eat your favorite food in moderation. In most days, keep your caloric intake low and eat healthy and organic foods as much as possible.

Do not allow yourself to get used to eating anything you please. When you get used to the bad habit, it is easier to go back to your lifestyle before the diet than to try the diet one more time. Always practice self-control. Look into the mirror and get inspired with what you have become after strictly following the diet.

You can also take a lot of pictures of yourself from the beginning of the diet until you have achieved your ideal weight. Look back into your old self – to how you looked before, especially at times when you are tempted to eat too much.

By measuring your progress, it will be easier for you to succeed in the diet and maintain the changes that you have attained. Set your expectations right and do not be too hard on yourself. You will reap more benefits from the diet if you will learn how to enjoy the process.

Chapter 8
Bonus Step- Myth Busting

When following any kinds of diet schemes, make sure that you always stay focused. It is typical to get ill advice and hear myths associated with the diet. Do your research first before you believe anything that you hear.

Here are the top myths about intermittent fasting and the truths behind them:

1. You will get fat when you skip breakfast often.

This logic comes from the belief that breakfast is the most important meal of the day. There are certain people who believe that the meal is special and should not be missed even when you are fasting. Missing breakfast often could trigger your cravings and hunger, which might result in weight gain.

There are studies, which proved that this is only a myth. Skipping breakfast will not result in weight gain. It actually depends on the individual characteristics of those who want to try the diet.

2. You can reduce hunger by eating often in small portions.

There are some people who can prove that this is true, but most dieters believe that this is a myth, especially the followers of IF. It is better if you will only eat whenever you feel hungry. Do not pop anything into your mouth to avoid feeling hungry even at times when you don't actually feel like eating.

3. Snacking is good for your health.

Snacking or eating often can increase your risk of certain health problems, especially when you snack on calorie-rich food. This will increase the stored fats in the liver, which will put you at a high risk of developing fatty liver.

There are certain studies, which proved that the habit increases your risk of having colorectal cancer. While your body can go on like usual for days even without food, it is not used to being fed constantly.

Fasting is actually healthier than eating often. It has good effects on your metabolic health and there are pieces of evidence linking autophagy to short-term fasting. Autophagy is a cellular repair process in which the cells use the stored protein in your system for energy. This leads to potential health benefits and gives you protection against aging, cancer, and Alzheimer's disease.

4. There is a limit in the amount of protein that your body can take per meal.

Some people claim that a human body is capable of digesting up to 30 grams of protein per meal. There are no studies that can prove this claim. The body is actually capable of taking in more than 30 grams of protein per meal. It is safe to consume more, especially if you need to meet the daily requirement for this nutrient.

5. The brain will not function well when you don't consume a good dose of glucose.

This is the reason why there are people who don't want to cut their carb intake. The system turns the carbs into glucose that the brain uses as fuel. Without a good supply of glucose, your body will turn to other sources that it can work on. In this case, it will make its own glucose through the process known as gluconeogenesis. This is used to supply the brain with fuel that can last for several hours. It doesn't happen all the time though because you have a stored glycogen in the liver.

When you fast for a longer duration and supply your system with very little carbs, the body will then burn fat and turn it into ketone. The brain will then use the ketone in the blood for fuel.

Take note that fasting is not suitable for everyone. There are those who feel hypoglycemic when they fast. If this is the case, it is recommended to eat small portions of meals throughout the day. You should seek your doctor's approval if you want to change anything about your diet.

6. Intermittent fasting is bad for your health.

IF is healthy and offers a lot of health benefits, but it is not suitable for everyone.

Make sure that you are fit to follow the diet before you commit to it.

Here are the frequently asked questions about the diet to help you understand more about the program:

1. Is intermittent fasting suitable for everyone?

The following are not suited to undergo this diet program:
- People who have recently undergone surgery
- Those who are under 18 years of age
- Those who are suffering from or have a history of serious mental health concerns
- Malnourished or underweight individuals
- Diabetics, especially the ones taking prescription medications
- People who are suffering or are recuperating from fever
- Pregnant women and breastfeeding mothers

- Individuals who are suffering from an eating disorder

Do not subject children and teens to fasting. It is better to make them wait until they become adults before they go into any kinds of diet. Healthy adults are suited to follow the diet, while it is not advised for old and frail individuals who often get sick.

2. Can anyone follow the IF program even though they don't have any weight problems?

Yes, you can follow IF as long as you are healthy and are not taking any kinds of medications. It offers more health benefits aside from weight loss. Even when you don't have a weight problem, you will still benefit from it as the diet aids in the repair and maintenance of the cells. This diet is also a good way to practice self-control.

3. Can you continue fasting even when you are sick?

It depends on your condition and how you feel. Listen to your body. If it is too sick to even move and feels very unwell, it is best to skip fasting. You need the nutrients that you can get from food in order to get well fast.

Fasting might worsen your health condition as it causes stress. The latter is the natural response of the body to speed up the repair process. It is easier to adapt to this kind of stress if you have enough energy from food.

4. How do you count calories when you are fasting?

It is easy as long as you plan your meals ahead of time. Follow recipes with nutritional information listed. This way, it will be easier for you to track your caloric intake. You can also check certain websites with available calorie counters that are free to use. As you go along the diet, you will have an idea about the nutrient content of each ingredient and how much are you allowed to consume to meet your daily nutrient requirement.

5. How hungry can you get?

It is only inevitable to feel hungry, but learn how to discern real hunger. There are times when the feeling will pass, which means that you were not really hungry but might only be craving for certain food. To get past this phase, you can keep yourself busy, go for a walk, or consume a calorie-free drink. Other people believe that you will starve when you fast, but this is only a myth. The truth is that the body boosts your metabolic rate at times when you take in a little amount of calories.

6. What are the side effects of the diet?

The first and obvious side effect of IF is hunger, especially in the beginning. This is normal and your system will eventually get used to it. You might also find it hard to sleep on an empty stomach at night. When this happens, you can have a light snack to satiate the hunger.

Keep yourself hydrated by drinking more water during the fasting hours. This will prevent you from having headaches and constipation. As long as you believe that this diet will work and you stay committed to it, you will experience fewer side effects and most of them are easy to handle.

You will feel shaky after fasting for several hours and this is only normal. Do not think too much about it. There are some people who faint from hunger but this is due to the fact that they contemplated a lot about the idea. Think positive and always cheer yourself. You are not bound to faint unless you are sick or diabetic.

7. Does it affect gout?

No. In fact, IF helps in reducing inflammation. Make sure that you stay hydrated all the time. It is also beneficial for the gout if you will avoid food that have high amounts of purine, such as cauliflower, liver, sardines, alcohol, lentils, and oatmeal.

Make sure that you are fit for the diet before you begin with it. Learn whatever you can about it in order to prepare for the changes. Commit to the diet and enjoy every step towards a healthier, more confident, and a better version of yourself.

Conclusion

Thank you again for downloading this book!

I hope this book was able to help you find the inspiration to follow this kind of diet and make this part of your lifestyle. I hope this has helped you on your journey towards the more confident and better version of yourself.

Finally, if you enjoyed this book, please take the time to share your thoughts and post a review on Amazon. It'd be greatly appreciated!

Thank you and good luck!

www.ingramcontent.com/pod-product-compliance
Lightning Source LLC
Chambersburg PA
CBHW060806260726
48660CB00002B/798